# LOW GI

## BELLY FAT DIET

The Flat Belly Action Plan

by Wesley Atkins

Published in Great Britain by:

LeadsClick
26 York Street
London
W1U 6PZ

© Copyright 2013 – Wesley Atkins

ISBN-13: 978-1493720781
ISBN-10: 1493720783

# Table of Contents

# INTRODUCTION:
# WHY YOU SHOULD READ
# EVERY WORD OF THIS BOOK

Have you tried many of the popular diet plans?

Have you become discouraged by your results that you fear you'll never be able to lose weight and keep it off?

If so, this book is for you.

Every week, some new diet book comes out with what sounds like a new twist on losing weight and feeling better. Most of them have their fifteen minutes of fame and then fade away into the half-price bookstores.

Let's face it - most diets are designed to get the weight off - but then what?

Once you stop using the diet it is very likely that the weight you lost will return, and often with a few extra pounds as a painful bonus. Most people end up feeling worse than they did before they started their new diet.

As such, many people simply give up in frustration and begin to accept their current weight and condition. This does NOT need to be the case for you anymore. Losing weight and keeping it off permanently does not need to be hit and miss.

Finally, there's a plan that has proven science behind it and a diet that you can use on a daily basis as long as you want - long-term. In fact, calling it a diet is doing it a disservice, as it becomes more of a lifestyle plan. It can fit into your daily routine easily and allows you to enjoy food and lose weight at the same time.

You've no doubt heard of - and perhaps tried - the cabbage soup diet, the Master Cleanser, and low fat diets. Generally speaking, you either;

**1.** Lose some weight but also lose your sanity, as life becomes an unbearable drudge of boring food, and you walk around in a state of constant hunger, or

**2.** You don't lose any weight because sticking to the restrictions of the diet is next to impossible.

In either case, these diets tend to leave you feeling bad about yourself. What you need is a new way of eating that is sustainable - a diet that doesn't feel like a diet at all! You need something that can truly be lived with day in and day out, all year long.

The perfect solution would be something that includes delicious foods and doesn't put any of your favourites completely off-limits. With this diet, you can stay healthy and slender without feeling deprived!

Eating during the day can certainly be enjoyable and it should be. It can also be health-oriented without being absurdly restrictive on the food choices.

Better yet, what is needed today is a way of eating that provides true energy - the kind of diet that will even give the middle-aged and elderly some of the energy they had when they were younger.

And what if this new diet (behaviour modification is a more accurate term) also made you healthier by strengthening your immune system, helping you to sleep better, and reducing silent inflammation?

## The Glycemic Index (GI) Diet

The Glycemic Index (GI) diet does all of those things and more. What is the GI diet? It's a diet based on foods with a low glycemic index, which refers to how a food affects your blood sugar. I'll explain that in more detail in a later chapter, but for right now, think of the GI diet as a moderate carbohydrate plan.

You're probably familiar with low carbohydrate (carb) diets. You've seen the advertisements: Lose Weight with the Low-Carb Diet, Gain Energy with the Atkins Diet, or even Get Your Six-Pack Abs with the South Beach Diet. With information overload like this, it can be hard to know which end is up.

The problem with most low carb diets (like Atkins) is that they are not suitable for athletes or even for those who exercise regularly. Why? The reason is simply that your body needs a certain amount of carbohydrates to fuel athletic activity.

The key here is to find the right amount of carbohydrates and which type are best for this purpose (there are some carbohydrates that should be avoided, but not all!).

Atkins is the most extreme low carb diet around - the induction phase allows you only 10% carbs. On this diet, if you exercised for no more than ten minutes, you'd experience a huge drop in your blood sugar levels (this is referred to as bonking by endurance athletes.)

The GI diet, on the other hand, strives to give you enough carbs without going too far in one direction or the other. You use a food's glycemic index rating (the degree to which it affects your blood sugar) to determine the best carbs to eat.

This plan is nothing new, however. The GI diet has been growing in popularity since 1981.

Why? ... Because it gets results.

Some of the results people see when using the GI diet include:

- Huge increases in energy
- They look better physically
- They feel healthier
- They lose weight
- They lower their blood sugar

The Atkins, Zone, South Beach, and other low carb diets are based upon a few of the same principles as the GI diet, but they go a bit too far in their restriction of carbs.

After reading this book, you'll have an understanding of how the GI diet works and will be able to make food choices that will keep your body energized and constantly burning fat.

Besides this, you will also understand which the best exercises to promote the fat-burning process in your body are, and you'll be able to combine this exercise with select foods for optimal health.

The key is to combine great tasting and healthy food choices with the correct amount of exercise, in order to ignite your metabolism and really start to burn the body fat and shed those unwanted pounds.

You'll learn how to look at any food or menu item and estimate its glycemic index off the top of your head. This will keep you choosing the best carbs to combine with proteins and fats so that you can make good split-second decisions about food. You'll then be knowledgeable enough to maintain a healthy lifestyle and live a life of abundant energy!

## Who benefits most from the GI diet?

The GI diet is aimed at people who want to lose weight,

but it's also the best fuelling method for athletes and sportsmen. Many people have commented that the diet itself has prevented or allowed them to recover from disease while others have reported a measurable increase in their energy.

Besides this, scientists and doctors have demonstrated how the GI diet is excellent for the control of diabetes in a number of case studies. For these reasons alone (the health benefits), it is worth switching to the GI diet, however there are of course the more obvious reasons.

When it comes to losing weight, nothing has been shown to work better than the GI diet because it's based on sound scientific principles. You can use the diet plans and meal plans to lose as much weight as you want.

For instance, the GI diet works even when people have a large amount of weight to lose. People have been known to lose **as much as 150 pounds** on the GI diet.

One of the huge benefits of the GI diet is that it allows you to lose weight while eating foods that are quite delicious and without suffering hunger pangs.

Once you begin to the use the diet and get accustomed to the new concepts and ideas, you will soon find yourself used to making a few simple calculations.

These are certainly not difficult or complicated as with many other diet plans. It is very simple and logical.

You'll also need to adjust your mindset to think of carbs

as fuel for activity. This is one of the big shifts that makes a huge difference for people on the GI diet.

Let's look at a quick example to explain this point;

If you work in an office and sit at a desk all day, then you won't need to eat very many carbohydrates at all. On the other hand, if you're going to play rugby for two hours, then you will need a higher volume of carbohydrates than most people.

In each of these cases, simple and specific calculations can be made to ensure you get enough fuel for activity without overloading and adding extra weight.

## How the GI diet came to be

The basic principles of the GI diet have essentially been around for centuries. It was the way many of our ancestors ate before factories began to over-process our packaged foods.

The current GI diet philosophy had its origins in the work of Dr. Robert Atkins, who wrote Dr. Atkins' New Diet Revolution in 1981. The diet was intended for weight loss, and it launched the Atkins diet, which is still very popular today.

When Dr. Atkins died recently, however, it was discovered that he had heart disease, which raised concerns about his diet plan. Science had already begun to believe that the Atkins Diet was too carbohydrate-restricted for long-term use and probably too high in fat.

Around the same time that Dr. Atkins' book came out, Dr. David Jenkins was studying the effects of carbohydrates on blood sugar and developed the Glycemic Index scale. What he discovered was revolutionary because it turned out that some sugary foods didn't affect blood sugar as much as some less sugary carbohydrates. This has to do with the composition of fat and protein. The rest is history.

Subsequent to Dr. Atkins' book, Dr. Barry Sears adapted the low carb philosophy to improve the performance of the Stanford University swim team. He called his system The Zone Diet and wrote Enter the Zone, the first of several books, in 1995. Critics complained that the Zone Diet was too complicated and required too much computation.

The latest entry into the low carb field is the South Beach Diet, which uses colorful photos of beach scenes to sell a diet that is more similar than any to the GI diet. But South Beach is also too restrictive, and besides, you don't need the latest diet craze. Contained in this book are all the no-nonsense facts you need to begin healthy low glycemic index eating, which is a sensible moderate carbohydrate diet approach.

# FREQUENTLY ASKED QUESTIONS (FAQ'S)

**Q:** Does the GI diet help you burn fat, especially belly and hip fat? Those are my worst areas.

**ANSWER:** Yes, this diet is designed to burn fat from your whole body including hip and belly fat. Insulin makes you store fat around your whole body and the GI diet burns fat by preventing insulin from flooding your system. The diet also allows glucagon to circulate, and glucagon stimulates fat burning.

**Q:** Is this just a fad diet?

**ANSWER:** No. In fact, it's actually not even a diet. Remember when your grandmother told you to eat all of your meat and vegetables because they were good for you? That's because she knew that protein plus some good fat plus low GI carbs were good for you, although she probably didn't say it in those words. The GI diet is simply sensible, healthy eating, which is why it's endorsed by many athletes and celebrities.

**Q:** Does the GI diet work for diabetics?

**ANSWER:** Since the GI diet is about lowering sugar consumption and reducing the possibility of a flood of insulin, it's a great diet to keep diabetes in check.

**Q:** Is this diet as hard to stick to as the Atkins Diet? I hated that one, and it gave me headaches and bad breath!

**ANSWER:** No, it really isn't as hard to stick to as the Atkins Diet. Low GI food is quite delicious, and you can have more carbs than on the Atkins Diet. Plus, people on the GI diet don't report headaches or bad breath.

**Q:** Will the GI diet ruin my metabolism like all the other diets I've tried?

**ANSWER:** Absolutely not. In fact, because of the thermogenic properties of low GI foods, it should increase your metabolism. Thermogenic means heat-producing, and it takes more energy for your body to burn low GI foods since they have a lot of fibre in them. Another way to increase your metabolism, of course, is to exercise more.

**Q:** Is this diet a cleanse?

**ANSWER:** It's not technically a cleanse, but it will probably make you healthier than any cleanse since you will be making lifelong dietary changes that are better for you.

**Q:** Does it work for any body shape, like apples or pears? For that matter, does it work for everyone?

**ANSWER:** Yes, it works for everyone because it works the way our bodies are designed to work. We have not evolved far enough to be able to handle simple carbohydrates, so we respond poorly to them. Anyone and everyone will benefit from the increased energy and lower body fat levels that the GI diet promotes.

**Q:** Is this one of those diets where you have success for a while and then just get stuck?

**ANSWER:** No, this is not the kind of diet that makes you plateau. Regular diets do that after about five weeks because you've lost only water and muscle during that time. Then, you get to the point where you can't lose much more muscle. It's really a false weight loss. The GI diet works because the combination of low GI foods and exercise cause your body to use muscle to burn fat.

**Q:** Is this the same thing as the South Beach Diet or the Atkins Diet? Those diets made me feel sick, and I almost went broke buying all the meat.

**ANSWER:** No, it's not the same. Those diets are about 80 to 90% protein. That amount of protein can actually be toxic to your kidneys. This is a sensible diet in which you consume moderate amounts of protein, low GI carbs, and good fats.

**Q:** Is this another one of those diets where you lose weight because the food tastes really bad, bland, and boring?

**ANSWER:** Not at all. The beauty of the low GI diet is that you can eat anything you want, in moderation. And adding a little healthy fat to low GI foods in the form of olive oil, macadamia nut oil, nuts, or avocados can make them taste very good. Did you know that most gourmet restaurants are actually serving low GI food?

**Q:** What about water? Do I have to drink eight glasses of water a day on this diet?

**ANSWER:** You should be drinking that much water all the time anyway, regardless of your diet. Here's the thing about water and weight loss: when you don't drink enough water, your kidneys have to work overtime to get rid of waste products. What do you do when you need help? You ask someone else for assistance. In this case, your liver pitches in for your kidneys to get rid of toxins. This is bad for the liver because it has to neglect its own work, which is metabolizing fat so that you can excrete it.

The bottom line is that water is necessary for your kidneys to function properly and for your liver to do its job of metabolizing fat. Also, if you exercise like I recommend, you will need to drink water to replace fat. Think of water as the lubricant that makes everything else in your body possible.

**Q:** If I lose weight on this diet, can I keep it off? If so, how do I go about that? That's always the hardest part.

**ANSWER:** Yes, you can keep it off. The GI diet isn't a temporary diet; it's a lifestyle modification. As long as you continue to eat low GI foods, you will keep your weight down. It's not hard once you get used to the change - low GI foods are fresh and delicious!

**Q:** Is this a low carb diet?

**ANSWER:** It's actually a low bad carb/moderate good carb diet. You need to minimize the high GI carbs you eat, and eat the moderate GI carbs sparingly. It's hard to go overboard with the low GI carbs since low GI foods have a lot of fibre that create a built-in mechanism against overeating - in other words, they're very filling.

**Q:** Are there such things as low GI desserts?

**ANSWER:** There are. Try a bunch of seedless grapes or half a mango with a scoop of low fat ice cream. You can also find low sugar or low carb desserts in the frozen foods section of most grocery stores. But with time, you'll be able to retrain your sweet tooth so that you won't crave sweets nearly as much.

**Q:** Are all low carb products low GI?

**ANSWER:** No, just because something is low carb doesn't mean it will also have a low glycemic index. This is something you have to watch. The carb that it does contain - even if it is a low amount - could be pure sugar. You need to carefully check ingredients.

**Q:** Are sugar substitutes safe to use?

**ANSWER:** Generally, no, since they're made from chemicals. The only two I know that are truly safe are Agave Nectar, which is made from the same plant they use to make tequila, and brown rice syrup. Both of these are moderate GI.

**Q:** How does adding vinegar or lemon juice lower the GI of a food?

**ANSWER:** They slow down the rate at which the carbohydrates in the food are absorbed into your bloodstream.

**Q:** How many calories should I be eating each day if I want to lose some weight in the form of fat?

**ANSWER:** If you're a woman, eat about 1,200 calories per day. For a man, eat about 1,500 per day. If you exercise - which you should certainly be doing - increase this number slightly. Make breakfast your biggest meal and dinner your smallest.

**Q:** I like to have a drink every now and then. Do I have to stop on the GI diet?

**ANSWER:** This is somewhat controversial, but no, I won't tell you that you can't have the occasional drink. Actually, a glass of red wine or a dark beer can be beneficial to your health. Please note I said ONE GLASS or ONE BEER, not 2 or 3 or 4 or more. When you do indulge, make sure you have a protein chaser and some decent fat to balance out the high GI carbs in the alcohol. The French know this, which is why they always pair wine with cheese.

**Q:** I'm a vegetarian. Will the GI diet work for me at all or should I look for something else?

**ANSWER:** Yes, it will work well for you. In fact, you

may benefit more from it than others, since a higher percentage of your diet comes from carbs. However, you will need to make sure you eat an adequate amount of protein, which you can do by combining foods such as beans and rice.

**Q:** I can't tolerate wheat and have to be on a low gluten diet. How would that affect the low GI plan?

**ANSWER:** There are plenty of other low GI flours you can use, such as spelt, quinoa, kamut, kashi, and others. Take a trip to your local health or natural food store to explore your options.

**Q:** Is the low GI diet safe? Does it have any bad side effects that could be harmful to my long-term health?

**ANSWER:** Yes, it is completely safe. There are no harmful side effects. In fact, there are many beneficial long-term effects such as loss of body fat, increased energy, improved sleep, decreased inflammation, better mood, and more.

**Q:** Do I need to add up all the low GI foods I eat every day and keep a list?

**ANSWER:** No, that's the beauty of this system. You can eat virtually unlimited amounts of low GI foods. Think about it - when was the last time you said, "Drat, I ate too many yams"?

**Q:** What are the best low GI foods for fighting cravings and hunger pangs?

**ANSWER:** Low GI foods combined with a little bit of healthy, monounsaturated fat will do the trick. For instance, try half an apple with a teaspoon of crunchy almond butter smeared on it, or eat a plum with 3 macadamia nuts. You could also have a piece of whole wheat toast with either ½ pat of butter or a teaspoon of olive oil.

# CHAPTER I:
# HOW SWEET:
# YOUR BLOOD SUGAR

In order to understand low glycemic index (GI) eating, you need to know a little bit about how your blood sugar levels operate.

Think back to the last time you ate candy, chocolates, or drank a soda like Coke (not the diet kind, but the real thing) for quick energy. It gave you a big energy boost for about 30 minutes, right? During those 30 minutes, your brain was working at top speed. You were talking fast and moving fast ... **but then ... plop!**

Your energy crashed again.

And this time you probably felt even more tired and lethargic than you did before you drank the soda. If you were at your desk, you probably longed for a nap because it was hard to keep your eyes open and stay focused. People often then have cravings for more candy or soda because the body is looking for the next quick energy fix.

Why this big energy crash?

It happened because candy bars and sodas contain a hefty dose of simple sugars. Simple sugars spike your blood sugar temporarily, causing it to soar for about 30 minutes. Then the beta cells in your pancreas determine that your blood sugar levels are too high, so your pancreas, which is in charge of regulating your blood sugar, releases insulin. <u>LOTS of insulin</u>.

As insulin floods your system, your energy sags, and you are now in a state of hypoglycaemia (low blood sugar.) This tends to keep you hungry, constantly looking for a way to keep your energy level up. But when you reach for the simple sugars again, the vicious cycle continues, and weight gain is the inevitable result.

So, simple sugars, eaten alone, will spike your blood sugar. Then, your body reacts, and your blood sugar PLUNGES. That's not good because in order to maintain your ideal weight and your mental edge throughout the business day, you need a sustainable level of energy that keeps your blood sugar on an even keel.

## The Secret Of High Energy All Day Long

Energy that spikes up and then shoots down is like starting a fire with crumpled newspapers. Sustainable energy, on the other hand, is like starting a fire with proper logs. The newspaper fire burns very fiercely for a short time, and then goes out. The log fire burns evenly for hours.

Your body needs an energy supply that you can rely on to

get you through the day. Thus, you need an energy source that won't turn your blood sugar into a roller coaster.

Now, I know what you're thinking. Why not just drink a Coke or eat a candy bar every 30 minutes? That way, just as my energy sags, it will pick back up again. This is a very bad idea for several reasons. For one thing, soda and candy bars have a lot of calories, and you'll gain weight - lots of it.

For another, sodas and candy bars also contain caffeine, so you'll have trouble sleeping. Even worse, new evidence is emerging that the consumption of too much sugar suppresses your immune system. In plain words, people who eat and drink lots of candy, pastries, and sodas get sick more often and may be prone to serious illnesses later in life.

So what foods provide you with a steady source of sustainable energy? Energy comes from carbs. Protein is used for muscle building and repair. Fat is used for energy storage.

## A Carb Is Not A Carb
## Is Not A Carb

The key thing to know is that not all carbs are the same. Some of them spike your blood sugar very quickly, others raise blood sugar more gradually, and still others ramp it up slowly and keep it at an even level for hours.

Complex carbs, such as broccoli or whole wheat pasta, raise your blood sugar gradually and keep it nice and even for hours. These are ideal carbs. So how do you know which carbs do what? By using the Glycemic Index (GI) chart.

The glycemic index ranks carbs based on their immediate effect on blood sugar levels (also called blood glucose levels.) Carbohydrates that break down quickly during digestion have the highest glycemic indexes. Your body's blood glucose response to these carbs is fast and high. Carbohydrates that break down slowly, releasing glucose gradually into the bloodstream, have low glycemic indexes. Your body responds to these in a much healthier way.

In the next chapter, we'll learn how all of this affects your health, energy levels, and body weight.

# Chapter II:
# The Glycemic Index (GI)

As we discussed in the last chapter, the glycemic index is a measure of how quickly a food or drink spikes your blood sugar, which depends upon how quickly the food turns into sugar after you eat it. This index runs from 1 to 100, and in this case, the lower the score, the better.

Foods and drinks that score low on the GI are healthy sources of steady, long-term energy. High GI foods and drinks, on the other hand, make your blood sugar behave like a bottle rocket - it shoots up, then crashes to earth. Simple table sugar, for example, has a GI of about 150!

The American Journal of Clinical Nutrition defines low glycemic as foods with a GI of less than 55, and high glycemic as foods with a GI of 70 or more. A GI value tells you how rapidly a particular carbohydrate turns into sugar. Mid-range GI foods, which have a rating of 56 to 69, can be included in your diet in moderation, and the great thing is that you can even have your favourite high GI index foods on occasion.

There are many reasons why you should strive to eat low GI foods. Here are a few:

- Gives a smaller rise in blood glucose levels after meals
- Keeps you feeling full longer
- Helps you lose weight
- Improves your body's sensitivity to insulin
- Can help to control diabetes
- Prolongs physical endurance

One of the other bad aspects of having your system flooded with insulin after a high GI meal is that insulin suppresses the release of glucagon in your body.

Glucagon is a hormone that pulls fat out of your cells and gives it to your muscles to burn for fuel. If you're trying to lose weight, you want glucagon circulating in your body. This is yet another reason why you **DON'T** want your system flooded with <u>insulin</u>.

Here's a pocket-sized chart of the GI of some common foods:

| Food | GI |
|------|-----|
| Plain Yoghurt | 14 |
| Fructose | 22 |
| Grapefruit | 25 |
| Apple | 38 |
| Orange Juice | 46 |
| Chocolate Bar | 49 |
| Cheese Pizza | 60 |
| Honey | 62 |
| Watermelon | 72 |
| French Fries | 73 |
| Bran Flakes | 74 |
| Pretzels | 83 |
| Baguette (bread) | 94 |
| Baked Red Potatoes | 95 |
| Tofu Frozen Dessert | 100 |

Are you surprised by what you see in this chart?

Most people are.

Who would have thought that something supposedly

good for you like a frozen tofu dessert could turn out to be such a culprit? And were you shocked to see the chocolate bar with such a low score, even borderline low GI?

You see, there are a number of common fallacies in circulation in the media and the magazines. While certain untruths are supported in order to sell more fad diets and foods, other become ingrained in people's mind, until they decide to question them.

## Take Fat Into Account

Here is another factor that you need to take into consideration. It's called fat. When fat is part of your meal or snack, it slows down the rate at which even simple sugars can hit your bloodstream. Fat acts as a type of control rod that regulates blood sugar. Thus, the chocolate bar scores only a 49 because of the fat it contains.

You can use this to your advantage if you want to work some high GI foods into your diet. Croissants have a GI of 67, which is borderline high. But if you spread some butter on them, you lower the GI because of the beneficial effects of the fat.

Of course, butter is a saturated animal fat, so you might want to find a healthier fatty spread. Olive oil is ideal since it is a monounsaturated fat (although it may taste better on French bread than a croissant).

This fat phenomenon also explains why baked red potatoes score 22 points higher than French fries on the glycemic index. The fries are cooked in oil, which adds fat. So, there's no reason to fear fat too much. However, it's still best to stick to monounsaturated fats like olive oil, avocados, macadamia nuts, Brazil nuts, almonds, hazelnuts, pumpkin seeds, cashews, etc.

And it's best to avoid saturated and trans fats, such as the fat found in margarine, shortening, fried foods, and most common snack foods, since they have been **linked to other health risks like heart disease**. You'll learn a bit more about fat in the next chapter.

## Making GI A Way Of Life

Later in this book, you'll find an index of the GI of many foods. You'll also find links to a larger index online. As you start using the GI, you'll start to memorize the score of your favorite foods.

Once you get a feel for GI, you'll be able to make decisions on the spot. You will ask yourself, what's the GI of that? And you'll also ask yourself how a particular food will make you feel for the next three to five hours. You'll make decisions based on fact and will be able to better control how you fuel your body each day.

# CHAPTER III:
# THE SCIENCE BEHIND GI

The GI concept has been around for a while, but not everyone understands the science behind it. It may sound complex, but stick with me. You'll soon understand how this powerful tool works.

## Fat is Not Evil!

First, something simple: Eating fat does not make you fat. I know we've all been programmed to believe this for the last 20-30 years. However, it's the companies who manufacture packaged carbohydrates like cakes and cookies who have been selling this message to increase their profit margins with products labelled as 'low fat'.

The truth is that some of these foods are worse for you than supposedly high fat foods.

**Case in point**: Studies show that people eat less fat today than ever before. Yet, obesity has never been more prevalent.

What DOES make people overweight? **INSULIN!**

Excess insulin makes you overweight and keeps you overweight by encouraging your body to store fat. It also drags down your metabolic rate and makes you feel tired and sleepy.

This means you need to think of food not so much in terms of nutrients, but more like a drug that has certain effects. Would you buy a drug that made you fat, sleepy, and gave you chronic inflammation? Of course not! If you eat a lot of fast food, this is essentially what you're doing.

A study at Children's Hospital in Boston on overweight teenage boys proved that a diet of mostly high GI foods caused them to eat more. Their appetites were simply greater because their bodies were always striving to get their blood sugar levels back up.

Again, your pancreas floods your system with insulin in response to high GI foods. It happens when you eat candy, non-diet sodas, pastries, cakes, and - believe it or not - even sports gels such as Gu or PowerGel, which claim to be good for you. Even many natural foods that you find in health food stores are high GI, such as honey, lemonade, and carob.

But there is hope! As people become educated about the dangers of high GI foods, action is being taken. A GI symbol program has been launched in Australia and New Zealand to help consumers easily identify foods that have been properly GI tested.

More information is available at:
http://www.gisymbol.com.au/

# Fat Facts

Oil that has been hydrogenated or partially hydrogenated is a trans-fat and should be avoided. The hydrogenation process adds shelf life to the food but negatively alters the chemistry of the fat. Trans fats are used in most common snack foods, and these fats are worse than pure butter or lard.

If a low GI food contains trans or saturated fat, for example, the sensible thing would be to put it on your list of very occasional foods. Eat mostly low GI foods with monounsaturated fats, and you will be in good shape.

If you're concerned about the calorie content of even monounsaturated fats, rest easy. There is much more to body chemistry than just the number of calories. Different types of foods are digested differently in the body, and this affects how the caloric content is absorbed. In other words, the type of food matters more than how many calories it contains. Stick with low GI foods and healthy fats, and you WILL lose weight.

# Facts on the Low GI diet

The glycemic index (GI) is a ranking of foods on a scale from 0 to 100 according to how much they spike your blood sugar levels after you eat them.

- The carbs that have a *high* glycemic index release their sugar into your bloodstream very quickly. This makes your blood sugar levels spike. Carbs with a low glycemic index release glucose more steadily over several hours. This helps to keep your blood sugar levels even.

- Pure glucose has a ranking of 100 on the glycemic index. Everything else is ranked in relation to glucose.

- High GI foods (above 70) include ice cream, croissants, raisins and other dried fruit, bananas, carrots, and watermelon. Moderate GI foods (50 to 70) include most types of pasta, baked beans, green peas, sweet potatoes, orange juice, blueberries, and rice. Low GI foods (under 50) include beans, cruciferous vegetables, high fibre/low sugar cereals, low fat unsweetened plain yogurt, grapefruit, apples, and tomatoes.

- Avoid foods that list sugar, high fructose corn syrup, or maltose as the first ingredient, as their GI is extremely high. (If sugar is listed first on an ingredients list, for example, that means there is more sugar in the item than anything else.) If you must have these foods, eat them infrequently and in small amounts.

GI ratings tell you how quickly foods are absorbed into your bloodstream. In this case, faster is not better!

# CHAPTER IV:
# THE GI DIET IN THE REAL WORLD

The GI index is great when you're making your meals at home. But what do you do when you're eating out with a group? How do you know what to eat and what to avoid?

I won't lie to you. It can be tough when you're trying to eat low GI foods in the real world. Most fast food restaurant items are loaded with simple sugars and saturated fat.

## The Lowdown On Low GI

The truth is that it's easiest to stick to the GI diet if you usually eat at home and pack a lunch to take to work. This will give you the most control over what you eat. But one of the toughest challenges for anyone who works in an office is the ritual of going out to lunch.

Eating dinner out is equally hard. You don't want your co-workers to think you're picky, but you'll have a devil of a time finding low GI foods at a place that specializes in hamburgers, fried chicken, or fish and chips. But it can be done!

# Guidelines for lowering your GI

- Increase your consumption of fruits, vegetables, legumes (peas and beans), nuts, and whole grains.
- Decrease your consumption of starchy, high-GI foods such as potatoes, white rice, and white bread.
- Decrease your consumption of sugary foods such as cookies, cakes, candy, and soft drinks.

# Eating Out

There are some times when you will need to eat away from home (unless you want to become totally constrained to your home). There are valid reasons for eating out and socialising with your friends and family.

Your diet should never be a restriction to your lifestyle – rather, it should enhance your lifestyle. As such, when you are eating out, there are a number of options you have available to you and you can take advantage of them. They may not be as good as having your pre-planned meals, but they will keep you from lapsing totally from your GI diet.

When eating at lunchtime you have a number of options:

# Sandwiches

If you are going to choose to eat a sandwich your best option is to choose a low GI takeaway sandwich. Ideally, in the best-case scenario, you should always make your own sandwiches before leaving for work or school, day trip etc.

Another couple of pointers here include:

Remember to always remove the top slice of bread or the top of the bread roll. Don't eat it, keep the sandwich or roll open faced. Also, ensure that the bread you are eating is wholemeal bread - this should always be possible as most places label their packaging and provide a wide variety of choices.

Always include at least three vegetables inside the sandwich. You could use tomatoes, cucumber, red or green peppers, lettuce, onion or bean sprouts. Remember that you can mix some of these up, so keep experimenting to see what fits your tastes best.

If you are going to use mayonnaise, then use low fat products. Alternatively you may want to use a salad dressing, but ensure this is low fat also.

If you are very rushed and can't take the time to make your own sandwiches, then here are some of the readymade options you can buy in your local city:

# Fast food restaurants

They have now started to introduce some low fat, healthier alternatives. They are also introducing menu items that have a low calorie count. One word of caution here: this is not a green light to start eating fast food on a regular basis. Such restaurants are known to add a lot of salt in order to make their product taste better. If you are able to cook your own meals, then please choose that option first.

**McDonalds** - although this fast food giant only has a small portion of food in the healthy category, it does seem to be growing, so if you are rushed choose one of the following options.

- Chicken tikka toasted deli sandwich - brown roll
- Chicken salad toasted deli sandwich - brown roll
- Grilled chicken ranch salad

**Subway** - this chain has the largest range of low fat, low calorie, and healthy choices in the fast food market. You have a number of options when you eat at Subway.

Their sandwich options (6 inch subs):

- Veggie delight
- Subway club
- Roast beef
- Roast chicken breast

- Turkey breast
- Turkey breast with ham

**Burger King** - Burger King were the last to bring a healthy alternative to the market, but they do now have some options for you to choose from:

- Spicy piri-piri chicken baguette
- Flame grilled chicken sandwich

# Tips when eating out on GI

- If the group insists on going to a hamburger joint, eat your burger open face by throwing away the top bun. You'll cut about 50% of the starchy carbs.
- Always order a large glass of water, even if it's mineral water, club soda, or fancy imported water - it doesn't matter. But avoid sodas - they're sugar traps, plain and simple.
- Skip desserts. If your friends tease you about it, have a cup of decaf coffee to be social.
- If you're at a fast food restaurant, order one of the entrée salads with meat in it, but avoid the taco salad, which has too many calories, carbs, and fats.
- For sandwiches, opt for chicken or fish, unless it's fried. Fried chicken and fish require a thick coating of white flour for breading, which raises the GI. Grilled chicken without the skin - eaten open face - is ideal!
- At dinner, skip the rolls or bread. They'll wreak havoc with your blood sugar.
- If everyone is drinking alcohol, you may have one drink as long as you eat sufficient protein with it. After one drink, switch to club soda.
- When picking side dishes at dinner, go for the veggies, and avoid baked potatoes or fries.
- Make sure you stay hydrated by drinking lots of water. Many times, a hunger pang is actually thirst in disguise.

- For a quick and low GI lunch, dash into a grocery store. Put together a salad from the salad bar, then go to the deli and buy 4 ounces of lunchmeat. Combine and enjoy!

Feeling good requires a bit of planning in a world that promotes unhealthy eating. While it can be a challenge to eat a low GI diet, the rewards are well worth it, and the alternative - low energy, excess weight, and illness - is simply not acceptable. Once you have created new habits, you'll no longer find the GI diet challenging. It will simply be a part of your routine like brushing your teeth in the morning.

# Chapter V:
# Meal & Snack Suggestions

For those times when you cook at home or prepare a lunch to take to work, here are some healthy suggestions that will keep you eating low GI foods. First, you'll need to shop differently, and you'll need to go to the grocery store more often. This is because the sugars in high GI foods have a preservative effect, giving these foods a much longer shelf life than fresh fruits, veggies, and meats. It sounds like a good thing, but it isn't. These sugars and preservatives are exactly what make these foods unhealthy.

So, it's definitely worth two or three weekly trips to the store to see an enormous change in your energy level. And don't worry, you won't be buying more groceries; you'll just be replenishing perishables.

## Skip the middle

There's an easy strategy you can use in the grocery store to stick with low GI foods. The stores stock high GI carbs in the middle aisles. Take a look next time you visit a grocery. What do they stock in the perimeter aisles? Meat, fresh vegetables, milk, delicatessen items, and the salad bar. Make the perimeter your new store, and simply stay out of the middle.

You may find that your grocery bill is slightly higher if you eat fresh veggies, fruits, and meats, rather than pancake mix, cereal, and bread. But then, these packaged products can often be more expensive than produce, and some people discover their appetite is lower when they stick to the GI diet. In short, it may even out in the long run.

If you do find that your grocery bill increases, you have to weigh that expense against your energy and your health. You may be preventing minor illnesses in the short term and serious illnesses in the long term. So, spending a little extra at the store will eventually save you money on medical care because you WILL be healthier! Think of it as a short-term investment in energy and a long-term investment in your health.

# Factors that affect the GI rating of a food:

- The more fibre a food contains, the lower its GI.
- Try not to cook foods too long. Longer cooking usually raises the GI. This is because cooking breaks down the beneficial fibre, and fibre slows down the rate at which a carb affects your blood sugar.
- If a low GI food is processed too much by the manufacturer, its GI will be higher.
- The addition of fat or oil to a food will lower its GI (although this is no reason to eat too much

saturated or trans-fat, which is simply unhealthy for you under any circumstances.)
- The addition of acids like lemon juice or vinegar will lower a food's GI.

## How often should you eat?

I recommend eating the standard three meals a day (breakfast, lunch, and dinner) with the addition of a mid-afternoon snack and a bedtime snack of about 100 calories each to keep your blood sugar from falling. And when you have a low GI snack before bed, you'll sleep better.

A good rule of thumb is to make breakfast the largest meal of the day, with the highest GI. I realize this is the opposite of what you've probably always been told, but a big breakfast will give you fuel for your day. Your smallest meal of the day should be dinner, since you're likely to be less active at night.

## Breakfast, Lunch & Snack Suggestions

Breakfast: Eggs, toast, juice

- 3 eggs, scrambled
- 1 slice white toast with ½ pat butter
- All-Bran cereal, 1 cup
- Skim milk, 8 ounces

Lunch: Sandwich, fruit & crackers

- Sandwich: 4 ounces of lunch meat on 2 slices of
- pumpernickel bread with 1 slice of cheese and mustard
- 1 medium apple
- 2 soda crackers

Snack: Apple and cheese

- ½ medium apple, raw
- 1 oz. cheese

Snack: Mini-sandwich

- ½ pita pocket
- Smear of sandwich spread
- 2 ounces sliced turkey
- Lettuce and tomato

# Sample Low GI Recipes

At the end of the book you will find over 25 recipes broken down into categories. For now, here's 3 to get your started.

## Pot Roast with Tomatoes

(Serves 4)

- 1 boneless bottom round roast beef (about 1-1/2 pounds)
- 1 small onion, minced (about 1/2 cup)
- 1 tablespoon Dijon mustard
- 1 (14.5 ounces) can diced tomatoes
- 1/2 teaspoon salt
- 1 teaspoon dried basil
- 1/8 teaspoon black pepper
- 3 tablespoons grated parmesan cheese

Preheat the oven to 350 degrees. Grease the roasting pan, and place the roast in the pan. Sprinkle the onions around the roast. Spread the mustard on top of the meat. Sprinkle the salt, pepper, and basil over the meat and onions. Top all with the can of diced tomatoes. Cover loosely and place in the oven. After about an hour of cooking, remove the cover from the roast. Sprinkle with the Parmesan cheese, and continue cooking uncovered for about another hour, until tender and the liquids are reduced in the pan.

## Cajun Chicken Casserole

(Serves 4)

- 1 whole chicken breast
- 2 tablespoons olive oil
- 1/2 cup chopped onion
- 2 cups cooked brown rice
- 1 can (14.5 ounces) diced tomatoes
- 4 ounces cream cheese, broken up into small chunks
- 1 cup Monterrey Jack or Colby cheese with jalapeno peppers, shredded
- 1 tablespoon Cajun seasoning
- Pinch of dried thyme

Grease a glass-baking dish, or spray with a non-stick spray. Preheat the oven to 325 degrees. Cut the chicken meat into bite-sized cubes, discarding any skin, fat, or bone. Heat the oil in a large skillet. Add the onions and sauté until translucent, but not browned. Remove from the heat. Add all remaining ingredients, except for about 1/2 cup of the pepper jack cheese. Toss together.

Pour into the baking dish, and top with the reserved shredded cheese. Bake for 30 minutes, until heated through and the cheese is melted.

## Blueberry Bran Muffins

(18 servings)

- 2 cups fresh blueberries
- 1-1/2 cups all bran cereal with extra fibre (contains less sugar)
- 1-1/2 cups plain soy milk
- 1 large egg
- 1/3 cup canola oil
- 3/4 cup Splenda
- 2 tablespoons freshly grated
- orange zest(peel)
- 1 teaspoon vanilla
- 1 cup whole wheat pastry flour
- 1 tablespoon baking powder
- 1 teaspoon cinnamon
- 3/4 cups chopped pecans

Wash the blueberries, and remove the stems. Place the berries on a paper towel to dry. Preheat the oven to 375 degrees. Grease your muffin tins, or line them with paper liners. In a large mixing bowl, mix together the cereal and the soy milk; soak this mixture for about 15 minutes. Stir in the egg, oil, Splenda, orange zest, and vanilla. In a separate bowl, combine the flour, baking powder, cinnamon, and nuts. Gently stir in the blueberries.

All at once, add the dry ingredients to the cereal mixture. Stir gently, just until blended. (Too much stirring destroys the light texture of muffins.) Spoon the batter into greased or paper-lined muffin tins. Bake the muffins for 25 minutes, until a cake tester inserted in the centre of one of the muffins comes out clean.

# CHAPTER VI:
# DESIGNING MEALS & SNACKS

So, how do you take what you've learned and create your own low GI meals and snacks? Well, it does require some thought. One thing that was eye-opening to me was to realize that you are what you eat, and with the food choices I had been making, I was cheap, easy, and fast -- not at all what I wanted to be!

Here are some general attributes of low GI foods to help you create meals and snacks that are anything but cheap, easy, and fast. Low GI foods are:

- Minimally processed - raw is best
- Whole grain
- High fibre
- Whole fruit instead of juice
- Not cooked or processed for very long

For breakfast, forget the orange juice and doughnuts, and go for things like eggs, Canadian bacon, whole grain breads, cereals or muffins, and skim milk.

At lunch, sandwiches can be okay if you choose whole wheat or whole grain breads and eat them open face with only one piece of the bread. Alternatively, a salad containing some meat and croutons or with a small roll is ideal. Choose vinaigrette over creamy salad dressings.

They're lower in fat, and the acid content of the vinegar will lower the dressing's GI.

When dinnertime arrives, think meat and vegetables, not pastas and breads, although a moderate amount of whole grain pasta or bread with butter or olive oil is alright. **Just don't overdo it!**

If you want to indulge in a high GI food, combine it with low GI foods. You will be creating a medium GI meal. Choose a wide variety of foods, and you will not only be healthier, but you'll enjoy eating much more. Discover new foods and new ways to prepare them. Cooking can be fun if you allow yourself to be creative and experimental.

# Sample Meal Plans

Use the sample meal plan below as a general guide for designing your own GI meals and weekly plans in advance. Having something set up ahead of time removes the excuses of snacking and choosing foods in the moment that are not good for you.

Planning is always the best option in order to stay with your new diet. Don't take this meal plan as the only thing available; once you have some experience with the new diet plan and the foods that you can use, you will then be able to substitute others in place of the ones you currently have.

You are able to replace other recipes and suggestions that you have already read inside this book. All of the suggestions are designed to be very quick to prepare and begin eating. And they are also designed to be enjoyable and satisfying. Hope you enjoy them!

Simply pick some of the choices below and order them into a set daily meal plan - make each day different to keep it interesting, and keep experimenting.

Remember the formula of the correct GI diet plan is to have breakfast, snack, lunch, snack, dinner and then another final snack. The list below takes this into account and enables you to make healthy choices from the many foods available.

Breakfast:

- Porridge
- Muesli
- Bran cereal
- Smoked salmon and scrambled eggs

Snack:

- Fruit yoghurt and almonds
- Carrots, cucumber, sliced pepper with light cheese
- Berry bars
- Light cottage cheese with fruit
- Cran-apple oatmeal bars
- Carrots, cucumbers, sliced peppers with hummus

Lunch:

- Warm spinach and bacon salad
- Cobb salad
- Open faced lean, thinly sliced chicken or turkey breast
- Sandwich with grainy mustard and salad
- Eggs and vegetables
- Open-faced tuna salad sandwich
- Salad
- Fruit yoghurt and almonds

Snack:

- Apple and almonds
- Orange cranberry bran muffin
- Mixed berry muffins
- 2 mini light babybel cheeses and a pear
- Fruit and almonds
- Berry bar and fruit

Dinner:

- Roasted chicken with tomatoes and asparagus
- Express cocoa spice rubbed grilled steak
- Sautéed greens with ginger
- Citrus fish steaks
- Speedy pork with lentils
- Chicken tarragon with mushrooms

- Express oriental salmon with leeks

Snack:

- Fresh berries tossed in lime juice and low fat crème fraiche
- Canned or fresh peaches with low fat cottage cheese, sliced pears with soya pudding
- Fruit salad with 2 medium scoops of low fat, low sugar ice cream
- Sliced pears with Soya pudding
- Fruit yoghurt and fresh berries
- Microwave crumble
- Raspberry fool

# Portion sizes

The idea of portion sizes in the GI diet is called glycaemic load and this gives you a more accurate idea of how certain foods behave in your body.

Glycaemic load is calculated by multiplying the food's GI by the carbohydrates per portion. You then divide the result by 100.

To represent the relationship between GI and GL, please see the table below.

| Value | GI | GL |
|---|---|---|
| High | 70 or more | 20 or more |
| Medium | 56-69 | 11-19 |
| Low | 55 or less | 10 or less |

**Remember this:**

The glycemic index value of a food tells you how rapidly a particular carbohydrate turns into sugar.

It doesn't tell you how much carbohydrates are in one portion of a particular food. Both the GI and the portion sizes are important to understand a food's effect on blood sugar. The glycemic index value alone does not give an accurate picture of the food. The glycemic load (GL) takes both the GI and portion size into account.

This is what you need to know in order to create your own recipes and meals. Use the GL to assure yourself that you are making the right choices of foods, and in the right portions. Some foods that are rated high on the GI may not have a negative effect on blood sugar levels, as long as the food has a low carbohydrate content.

For example carrots have a GI of 92, which seems very high, but a 100g serving has only 5.2g of carbohydrate resulting in a very low GL of only 4.3. This means carrots also have a large amount of water, dietary fibre, and a small amount of protein.

# CHAPTER VII:
# GOOD CARBS, BAD CARBS

What's the difference between a good carb and a bad carb? As we've said, the good ones will provide you with a steady source of sustainable energy for hours. The bad ones will spike your blood sugar sky-high for about 30 minutes, then bring it crashing back down to earth.

Then, there are the carbs in between. If good carbs are like a green traffic light, and bad carbs are a red light, then the ones in between (which we will call moderate carbs) are yellow lights. In other words, proceed with caution.

As you know, good carbs are low on the glycemic index with a GI of less than 50. In general, these are whole grains, multi-whole grain bread, vegetables, and some fruits. The closer a carb is to its natural, unrefined, unprocessed state, the better it is for you.

Bad carbs are high on the GI scale - above 70. They include simple sugars like dextrose, sucrose, high fructose corn syrup, and fructose itself. Many carbs start out as moderate or good carbs but end up as bad carbs because manufacturers process and refine the living daylights out of them.

Case in point: sugar. Raw sugar cane isn't all that bad for you; it's a moderate carb. But when it's refined into table sugar, the GI shoots up into the high region. The same thing is true of raw wheat. It's a complex carb that's good for you. But when a manufacturer crushes, sifts, and refines it into white flour, the GI increases greatly.

# Five Star Carbs

So, what should you look for? Raw, unprocessed carbs like whole grains, vegetables, and fruits are best. The only downside is that these foods do take time to prepare and cook. If you find yourself in a time crunch, and you don't have time to cook, you can buy your carbs in the store, pre-packaged.

When you buy pre-packaged carbs, however, be on the lookout for too much processing or added ingredients that increase the GI index. If you don't have time to cook oatmeal from scratch, for example, read the ingredients before buying those little packets that just require the addition of hot water. If the first, second, or third ingredient is sugar or some form of it like high fructose corn syrup, it contains much too much sugar. Find another brand!

Sodas have a very high GI. Almost all of them list high fructose corn syrup as the first ingredient. If you must have the occasional soda, make it very occasional.

Now, as I've said, you CAN make a bad carb good by adding some fat or protein to it. You can't do this with all bad carbs though, since adding fat or protein doesn't help when it comes to straight sugar. But if you crave French bread made from refined white flour, go ahead and have a small slice or two with some heart-healthy olive oil. The oil combined with the bread will lower the GI of the two together.

## Low Glycemic Index Foods

(GI is 55 or less)

Eat some at every meal

- Skim milk
- Plain Yogurt
- Soy beverage
- Apple/plum/orange
- Sweet potato
- Oat bran bread
- Oatmeal (slow cook oats)
- All-Bran
- Converted or Parboiled rice
- Pumpernickel bread
- Al dente (firm) pasta
- Lentils/kidney/baked beans
- Chick peas

## Medium Glycemic Index Foods

(GI is 56-69)

Eat these in moderation

- Pineapple
- Raisins
- New potatoes
- Popcorn
- Split pea or green pea soup
- Brown rice
- Couscous
- Basmati rice
- Shredded wheat cereal
- Whole wheat bread
- Rye bread

# High Glycemic Index Foods

(GI above 70)

Eat these sparingly

- Watermelon
- Banana
- Dried dates
- Instant mashed potatoes
- Baked white potato
- Parsnips
- Rutabaga
- Instant rice
- Corn Flakes
- Rice Krispies
- Cheerios

- Bagel, white
- Soda crackers
- Jellybeans
- French fries
- Ice cream
- Digestive cookies
- Table sugar (sucrose)

How to use these tables depends on your gender and bodyweight. But generally, you should eat low GI foods at every meal and every snack. You can eat moderate GI foods once per day, and you may indulge in high GI foods once or twice a week.

## Sample Day On
## The Low GI diet

Breakfast:

Scrambled eggs consisting of 3 egg whites and 1 yolk
½ cup of all-bran cereal
skim milk

Lunch:

Small tuna salad sandwich, whole wheat bread
1 cup plain yogurt
½ apple

Afternoon snack:

1 strip beef jerky
orange.

Dinner:

6 ounces of broiled salmon with lemon dill butter
1 cup of steamed vegetables. Broccoli / green beans.
3 ounces of mashed sweet potatoes dressed with olive
oil and rosemary.

Bedtime snack:

½ cup plain yogurt
2 ounces of blueberries.

# Your Kitchen and Low GI Eating

Equip your kitchen with a good cutting board, a high-quality chef's knife, and some decent non-aluminium pots and pans. If you can take the extra time and effort to prepare foods that are minimally processed and not refined, you will find it easier to eat low GI foods. This means cutting up vegetables, simmering oatmeal, baking breads from whole wheat grains, and things like that. The best reward for your efforts will be delicious, fresh food.

**Tip:** An electric bread maker is a great way to include whole grain, low or no sugar breads into your diet. It's quick and easy to place the ingredients into the machine, and set the timer to begin baking in time for you to awaken to the smell of fresh bread.

When you purchase whole grain flours, however, keep them in the refrigerator. The natural oils in unrefined flour will become rancid without proper refrigeration.

| Excellent Snack Foods | Excellent Oils |
|---|---|
| Fresh Fruit | Extra Virgin Olive Oil |
| Chopped Vegetables | Flax Seed Oil |
| Nuts | Canola Oil |
| Seeds | Walnut Oil |
| Plain Yoghurt | Wheatgerm Oil |

# Directory of GI Foods

The glycemic index range is as follows:

- Low GI = 55 or less
- Medium GI = 56 - 69
- High GI = 70 or more

The numbers to the right of the foods are the glycemic index of the foods. This should give you a clear idea of which foods to eat and those to avoid, or eat very sparingly.

A great printable chart for High, Medium and Low GI

Foods can be found on the GI diet Guide website, a great resource, found here:

http://www.the-gi-diet.org/lowgifoods/

# CHAPTER VIII:
# EXERCISE IS NOT OPTIONAL

Dieting alone is not an effective way to lose weight, even if it's an excellent diet like GI. Why not? Because dieting without exercise actually lowers your metabolism. This is why many people gain back the weight they lost - plus some. Lean muscle is what burns fat.

If you don't work out, you won't have much lean muscle to burn fat. And if you don't have much lean muscle, you won't have what you need to burn fat - pure and simple. Think of fat as gasoline and your muscles as engines. If you really want to burn a lot of gas, you need more and bigger engines. Thus, you need to build muscle. How do you build muscle? There are several ways.

## Find a Fun Aerobic Exercise

What form of aerobic exercise should you do? The one you enjoy most! That way, you are more likely to stick with it. The most efficient aerobic exercise is running, since it burns the most calories per hour, but if you don't like running or if you have bad knees, there are plenty of viable alternatives.

To build cardiovascular fitness and improve general muscle tone, you need one half-hour of aerobic exercise four times per week. This can include brisk walking with weights, running, cycling, rowing, swimming, or any kind of cardiovascular fitness classes. Aerobic exercise also keeps your heart and lungs in good shape. Be moderate when you begin, however, and gradually work yourself up to more challenging exercises. It's best to do no more than one hour of aerobic exercise at a time because more will just tear down that precious muscle tissue that burns fat.

**Note:** A special word to women: when I talk about lean muscle, I'm not recommending you bulk up like a bodybuilder. I'm referring to a modest amount of lean muscle that gives you a very pleasantly toned and sculpted look.

## The Joys of Multisport

My personal favorite aerobic exercise is multisport. This is a growing trend that has spawned two very popular endurance sports: the triathlon and adventure racing. If you've been stuck doing one sport for a long time, you can reenergize your body, mind, and spirit by going multisport.

What does multisport mean? At its most general, it means doing more than one sport. For instance, mountain bikers who are also trail runners are multisport athletes. But today, multisport commonly means the triathlon, which generally entails swimming, road cycling, and road running. Sometimes swimming is left out, so the event is then called a duathlon. There are also a growing number of off-road triathlons and duathlons.

Some say adventure racing - the wild and wooly distant cousin of the triathlon - is growing even faster than triathlons. The specific events involved in an adventure race can vary, but there are almost always three core disciplines: mountain biking, trail running or hiking, and paddling a canoe or kayak.

You don't have to compete in triathlons or adventure races in order to get in on the fun and fitness involved in multisport training and reap the benefits of burning calories and conditioning your muscles. So how do you juggle three sports within one short week?

The key lies in realizing that you don't have to train in each sport three or more times weekly. When you do multisport, there's a cross-training effect. For instance, cycling benefits running and vice versa. And some sports, such as swimming and paddling, may be seasonal for all but the most hard-core athletes.

A typical multisport week in February might look like this:

- Monday - Run intervals.
- Tuesday - Cycle for an hour at a moderate pace.
- Wednesday - Swim for thirty minutes.
- Thursday - Take the day off.
- Friday -- Run two to four miles.
- Saturday - Cycle three hours on a group ride.

- Sunday - Rest or lift weights.

Here's an alternative schedule:

- Monday - Play tennis.
- Tuesday - Paddle on a lake.
- Wednesday - Take a Pilates class (Pilates is a specialized and popular program of mat exercises and machines which focuses on strengthening the abdominal muscles.)
- Thursday - Lift weights.
- Friday - Take the day off.
- Saturday - Play tennis.
- Sunday - Take a Pilates class.

The general idea is that you work out five or six days a week and spread the workouts among two, three, or more sports. If you're younger than 40, you can probably work out twice a day, but don't try to do that every single workout day.

## What are Brick Workouts?

Bricks are workouts in which you do more than one sport in the same workout. As an example, you might cycle for an hour, then hop off and, as quickly as you can, change shoes and run for 30 minutes. This works your muscles in new ways and will tire you out considerably, so ease slowly into bricks. A brick once a week is plenty to start with.

If you decide you'd like to compete, you'll want to add some brick workouts to your routine, but wait until you've been into the multisport training groove for about six weeks.

Even if you don't compete, a brick can be fun, calorie-consuming, and therapeutic. One of my personal favourite bricks is mountain biking, followed immediately by swimming. Studies have shown that immersing yourself in cold water makes you less sore after a workout because it flushes waste products out of your muscles.

What if it's a cold and rainy day and you don't want to work out outdoors? A Pilates or cardiovascular workout class at the gym followed by a half-hour of spinning would be an excellent brick. You could also run on the treadmill and follow it up with a 15-minute swim in the gym's lap pool.

Follow a few general principles during cold weather like making sure you take off one or two days a week, and refrain from training in each sport more than three times weekly. This will have you in the multisport groove by the time the warm weather hits, and then you can tackle the triathlons and adventure races.

# The Importance of Weight Training

I recommend adding a bit of resistance work or weight training to your aerobic exercise regimen. If you've never worked with weights, start by lifting light weights (1-5 pounds) twice per week. On one day, lift for your lower body, and on the other day, lift for your upper body.

Select exercises that are compound in nature, meaning that they use many major muscle groups. What you don't want to do are isolation exercises that just work one muscle, such as bicep isolation curls.

# Recommended Exercises (Lower Body)

**Squats** - Only do full squats if you are under 35 and have good knees. Do not bounce when you do squats. If you have any knee problems or are over 35, do partial squats (your thigh does not descend to where it is parallel to the floor.) Squats strengthen your lower quadriceps (muscles in your thighs), upper hamstrings (muscles in the back of your legs), and gluteals (muscles in your buttocks.)

**Leg curls or lunges** - These exercises strengthen your hamstrings.

**Deadlifts** - Keep your back flat and look up as you do these lifts, which strengthen your back and gluteal muscles.

**Crunches** - or other abdominal exercises to strengthen your abdominal muscles, which in turn strengthens your back.

**Calf raises** - These strengthen your soleus muscles which lie underneath your calves.

**Foot flexes** - These are the opposite of calf raises and strengthen the tibialis anterior muscles in your legs.

# Recommended Exercises (Upper Body)

**Bench press** - This exercise is often regarded as the king of upper body exercises. Don't bounce the bar off your chest though, as it's dangerous, and you won't strengthen the muscles in the bottom part of the range. The bench press strengthens your chest muscles, the front of your shoulders, and your triceps (the muscles at the back of your upper arms.)

**Rowing exercises** - either seated or bent over - These are great for strengthening your upper back.

**Lat pull downs or chin-ups** - These exercises strengthen the lateral back muscles, giving you a nice V-shape.

**Presses** - either behind the neck or in front, with barbells or dumbbells - These exercises strengthen your shoulders.

**Shrugs** - These strengthen the trapezius muscle, which runs along the shoulder from the neck.

**Bicep curls** - These are done with a barbell or cable bar and strengthen the bicep muscles in the upper arm.

**French press or cable push-downs** - These are great tricep strengtheners.

# How Many Repetitions?

There are many ways to do weight exercises. One thing you want to avoid is doing the same number of repetitions for more than a month. Try this:

- One set of 30 repetitions of each exercise for four weeks.
- Two sets of 15 repetitions for four weeks.
- Three sets of 5 repetitions for two weeks.
- One week where you do one set of 30, one set of 15, and one set of 5.
- Then take a full week off and start the cycle again.

The most important thing to remember as you develop your exercise routine is to find sports, classes, and exercises that you enjoy. If it's a drudge, you won't do it - pure and simple. Keep looking until you find activities that are fun for you, and remember that any exercise will become easier as you get more in shape. So, don't give up too quickly!

## Sample Body Conditioning Routines

Routine I

- 25 normal pushups
- 25 sit-ups
- 25 squats with feet flat
- 25 star jumps

- 25 v-ups

This routine should only take about 5-10 minutes to complete. It is very simple but hard work if you keep the intensity high. You can repeat this routine 3-5 times as you get more and more proficient.

Routine II

- 10 mins skipping (1 set)
- 25 lunges (1-3 sets)
- 10 pullups (1-3 sets)
- 25 pushups (1-3 sets)
- 15 dips (1 set)
- 25 crunches (1-3 set)

Routine III

- 20 pushups variation (1-3 sets)
- 15 mountain climbers (1-3 sets)
- 25 high knees (1-3 sets)
- 30 squats (1-3 sets)
- 15 lying side crunch (1-3 sets)

Remember that it is a good idea to change your routine and bring in new movements in order to work your body from different angles and avoid training plateaus.

# CHAPTER IX:
# PULLING IT ALL TOGETHER

You now have all the tools you need to eat healthier by lowering the glycemic load of your daily food and drink intake. I promise you that your energy will increase, you'll feel and look healthier, and you will have a new and improved outlook on life. Many people report that the diet even improves their mood. What's more, you'll probably lose weight!

One thing I want you to keep in mind is the old saying that it takes 30 days to change a bad habit. The opposite is also true: it takes about 30 days to firmly establish a good habit. So, any change requires a commitment. Right here and right now, promise yourself that you will stick with the GI diet for at least 30 days. After that, you won't want to do anything else.

## The Proof is in the Results

I guarantee you that if you stick with this diet faithfully for 30 days, and you exercise, including aerobic and a bit of weight training, you will:

- Lose body fat, especially stubborn belly, bottom, and hip fat.
- Increase your energy level substantially.

- Look and feel much better (and receive compliments from your friends).
- Enjoy life more.
- Be able to enjoy the foods you love in moderation and discover new foods and tastes that will delight you. (You may even discover a hidden talent for cooking!)
- Control your diabetes, if you have it.

The low GI diet is not a fad. It's a permanent behaviour modification plan, and it hearkens back to the way we were meant to eat before factories began to over process foods, adding so many sugars to preserve the shelf life of packaged high carbohydrates.

# Where To Go From Here...

At this stage in the diet transformation process, you should have seen many amazing results both in your physical body shape and also in your health. You will probably look and feel a lot better about yourself. Your energy levels should have also risen by leaps and bounds.

All of these benefits are very positive, but the question for most people is where to go from this point forward.

Well, first you should congratulate yourself for getting this far, because most people never will. If you have stuck to the diet plan, then you will have reached your target weight, and you will feel as though you have a new lease of life. In only a few short weeks, you will have totally transformed yourself, and probably gained more confidence than you thought possible.

However, this does not mean you should rest easy and take a break.

Remember that this is a lifestyle choice and you can support yourself in that choice. Keep your goals clearly in mind and be clear about your reasons for making this change.

Not only that, but this stage will also see you move from a weight loss plan to a weight maintenance plan. This change can cause some people to become unclear and gradually they will start to revert back to their old habits and weight, but this is not going to happen to you - **if you follow this advice.**

Remember, this is going to be the phase you can follow for the rest of your life. In order to stay on course, you are going to make the diet and lifestyle very attractive to follow. This is the big key that most people miss.

Most people think that the goal has been reached and it seems more attractive to go back to the old ways than it does to maintain their new healthy body and lifestyle. Here is the reason why so many people abandon their weight loss goals and return to their previous unhealthy, overweight selves. Or in some cases, they end up even worse off than when they started.

Can you relate to that?

I'm sure you have either seen or experienced this for yourself. It is commonly called the yo-yo effect in dieting and can actually cause severe health problems in the long term.

Remember that the keys are to stick to your system that you have built up over the last few weeks. If you need to make any changes or feel inclined to do so, then do things one at a time.

Change aspects of your diet slowly and measure them.

Remember and understand that the nature of your body and metabolism has now become used to needing less calories than you used to digest. Your body is now far better at burning up calories as your metabolism has increased in capacity.

Because you don't need as many calories to function effectively throughout the day anymore, any big changes will see the weight come back. If this starts to happen, then look at your diet system and return to your weight loss phase diet for a time. Keep track of the changes and you will soon see which foods and in which quantity are acceptable to eat.

Keep the following equation in mind:

In order to maintain your weight - you must balance the calories (energy) that you digest with the amount of energy you expend each day.

I urge you to begin on the GI diet plan today while you

feel inspired to do so. It's never too late to experience the high energy you are meant to feel, as well as your ideal weight and optimal health. This is what can be yours when ... **You take action!**

# CHAPTER X:
# DELICIOUS LOW GI RECIPES

## Breakfast Recipes

### Porridge

Preparation Time: 15 minutes

Serves: 4

Ingredients:

- 1 cup rolled oats
- 2 1/2 cups water
- Teaspoon salt
- 1/2 cup sultanas
- 2 bananas, sliced
- Pinch of salmon

Instructions:

1. Place oats, water, salt, bananas and cinnamon in a saucepan. Bring to a boil then simmer until all the water has been absorbed.
2. Stir frequently.
3. Pour porridge into bowls. Add cold milk and brown sugar if desired.

## One-Pan Summer Eggs

Preparation Time: 20 minutes

Serves: 2

Ingredients:

- 2 large zucchinis, chopped
- 200 grams cherry tomatoes, halved
- 2 eggs
- 1 tablespoon olive oil
- 1 clove garlic, crushed
- Fresh basil leaves
- Salt and pepper

Instructions:

1. Heat oil in a frying pan over medium fire.
2. Cook zucchinis in oil, stirring frequently, until tender. Stir in tomatoes and garlic. Cook for a few more minutes until tomatoes are soft. Add salt and black pepper to taste.
3. Make two empty spaces in the pan for the eggs. Crack eggs over the spaces and cover pan until eggs are cooked to your liking.
4. Sprinkle a few fresh basil leaves and serve.

## Zucchini Fritters

Preparation Time: 25

Serves: 6

Ingredients:

- 1 large zucchini, grated
- 1 small onion, chopped
- 1 clove garlic, minced
- 3 eggs, beaten
- 1/2 cup Romano cheese, grated
- 1 tablespoon parsley, chopped
- 1 cup milk
- 2 cups whole wheat flour
- 2 tablespoons olive oil
- Salt and pepper

Instructions:

1. Mix zucchini, onion, garlic eggs, cheese parsley, milk and flour in a large bowl. Add salt and pepper to taste.
2. In a large pan, heat 1 tablespoon olive oil over medium fire. Place identical-sized chunks of batter into the oil and fry. Flatten with a spatula.
3. Cook fritters until the centre appears golden brown. Turn and cook on the other side.
4. Do the same with the remaining batter. Add more oil as needed.

# Strawberry and Banana Wholemeal Muffins

Preparation Time: 35 minutes

Serves: 12

Ingredients:

- 1 3/4 cups wholemeal flour
- 250 grams strawberries, fresh or frozen
- 3 ripe bananas, mashed
- 1/2 cup applesauce
- 1 cup dark brown soft sugar
- 2 eggs
- 1 teaspoon vanilla essence
- 3 teaspoons cinnamon
- 1 teaspoon bicarbonate soda
- 3 tablespoons vegetable oil

Instructions:

1. Preheat oven to 190C.
2. Grease a 12-cup muffin tray or line with muffin paper cups.
3. Combine eggs, bananas, applesauce, brown sugar, oil and vanilla essence in a blender. Whip together until slightly lumpy.
4. Mix flour, cinnamon and bicarbonate soda in another bowl. Fold into banana mixture until flour is just slightly moist.
5. Add strawberries into the mixture and fold.
6. Use an ice cream scoop to place equal amounts of batter into the muffin tray.

7. Bake for 20 minutes.
8. Place muffins in a cooling rack before removing from tray.

## Apple and Cinnamon Muesli Bars

Preparation Time: 45 minutes

Serves: 14 bars

Ingredients:

- 1 cup rolled oats
- 1/2 cup All-Bran
- 1 1/2 cups Rice Bubbles
- 1/2 cup wholemeal flour
- 1 cup applesauce, unsweetened
- 3/4 cup brown sugar
- 1/2 coconut
- 1 cup dried apple, diced
- 1 tablespoon honey
- 125 grams butter
- 2 teaspoon cinnamon

Instructions:

1. Preheat oven to 150C.
2. Lightly grease a Swiss roll tin or line with baking paper.
3. In a small saucepan, cook butter, sugar and honey over low fire. Stir constantly until sugar melts. Set aside and let cool.
4. Combine oats, All-Bran, Rice Bubbles, flour, brown sugar, coconut, apple and cinnamon in a mixing bowl. Mix well.
5. Add applesauce into butter mixture and stir until well-blended.

6. Pour liquid mixture into the dry ingredients and mix.
7. Transfer batter into the Swiss roll tin and press down firmly.
8. Bake for 30 to 40 minutes until golden bar.
9. Place tin in cooling rack.
10. Cut into rectangular pieces of identical size.

Tips:

- Let the mixture bake longer if you want crunchy bars. For a chewier texture, bake less.
- If you're having crunchy bars, cut them while warm. Waiting for it to cool will result in flaky muesli bars.
- To make your own apple sauce, dice two large apples and stew over low fire for 1 hour. Place the lid and do not add water or sugar.

# Oat Pancakes with Banana

Preparation Time: 55 minutes

Serves: 4

Ingredients:

- 2 cups buttermilk
- 1/2 cup rolled oats
- 2/3 cup wholemeal flour
- 2/3 cup plain flour
- 1 1/2 teaspoons baking powder
- 1/2 teaspoon bicarbonate soda
- 1/2 teaspoon cinnamon
- 1/4 cup wheat germ
- 2 eggs
- 1/4 cup brown sugar, firmly packed
- 1 teaspoon vanilla essence
- 1/2 cup maple syrup, warmed
- 2 medium bananas, sliced

Instructions:

1. Combine oats and buttermilk in a small bowl and set aside.
2. Sift wholemeal flour, plain flour, baking powder, bicarbonate soda and cinnamon into a large bowl.
3. Add wheat germ and husks from wholemeal flour.
4. Place eggs, sugar, oil and vanilla essence in a medium bowl and whisk.

5. Pour buttermilk mixture into the egg mixture and stir.
6. Add the liquid ingredients into the flour mixture and fold with a rubber spatula until the flour is just moistened.
7. Coat a non-stick frying pan with cooking spray. Heat pan over medium fire.
8. Scoop 1/4 cup of batter into the frying pan and cook for 2 to 3 minutes or until bottom side is golden brown and top side forms small bubbles. Turn pancakes and cook the other side for 1 to 2 minutes.
9. Repeat until all batter is cooked. Place pancakes in a 90C oven to keep them warm.
10. Top with banana slices and drizzle with warm maple syrup before serving.

Tips:

For left overs, wrap pancakes in individual plastic wraps and place in freezer. Take them out and reheat in an oven toaster as desired.

# Lunch Recipes

## Maple-Roasted Chicken and Pumpkin Salad

Preparation Time: 55 minutes

Serves: 4

Ingredients:

- 800 grams butternut pumpkin, peeled and chopped
- 600 grams chicken breasts fillets
- 100 grams spinach and rocket salad mix
- 1/2 cup walnuts
- 2 tablespoons maple syrup
- 1 tablespoon olive oil
- 1 red onion, sliced thinly

For dressing:

- 2 tablespoons olive oil
- 2 tablespoons apple cider vinegar
- 2 teaspoons maple syrup
- 1 teaspoon wholegrain mustard

Instructions:

1. Preheat oven to 220C.
2. Lightly grease a baking pan or line with non-grease baking paper.
3. Mix pumpkin, oil and syrup in a mixing bowl and toss. Add salt and pepper to taste.
4. Place pumpkin mixture in a single layer on baking pan and bake for 20 to 30 minutes or until pumpkin is tender. Add walnuts during the last 8 minutes of baking.
5. Spray a frying pan with cooking oil and heat over medium-high heat.
6. Cook chicken for 6 to 7 minutes on each side or until chicken is brown.
7. Remove chicken from pan and let stand on a plate. Slice chicken into strips.
8. To make dressing, pour oil, vinegar, syrup and mustard in a jar. Close the lid tightly and shake well.
9. Place pumpkin mixture, chicken, dressing and onions in a large salad bowl and toss. Add more walnuts if desired.

## Chicken Coleslaw Sandwich

Preparation Time: 15 minutes

Serves: 2

Ingredients:

- 60 grams chicken, shaved
- 1/2 cup cabbage, shredded
- 1 small carrot, grated
- 1 green onion, sliced
- 2 tablespoons mayonnaise
- 1 teaspoon lemon juice
- 4 baby cos lettuce leaves
- Salt and pepper
- 4 slices wholegrain bread, buttered

Instructions:

1. Place cabbage, carrot, onion, mayonnaise and lemon juice in a large bowl and mix well. Add salt and pepper to taste.
2. Put 2 lettuce leaves over two slices of bread. Top with coleslaw and chicken. Place 2 more lettuce leaves for each sandwich and top with the remaining slices of bread.
3. Cut sandwiches in two and cover with plastic wrap.

## American-Style Mac n' Cheese Frittatas

Preparation Time: 45 minutes

Serves: 6

Ingredients:

- 120 grams macaroni pasta
- 80 grams cheddar cheese, grated
- 250 grams corn kernels, rinsed and drained
- 1 medium carrot, peeled and grated
- 1 small red capsicum, halved, deseeded and chopped
- 1/2 cup milk
- 7 eggs, whisked lightly

Instructions:

1. Cook pasta in a pot of boiling water until al dente. Drain and place under cold, running water to cool. Drain well.
2. Preheat oven to 180C and lightly grease six non-stick muffin trays.
3. Mix pasta, cheese, corn, capsicum and carrot in a large bowl.
4. Scoop pasta mixture into muffin trays.
5. Beat egg and milk in a bowl and pour over pasta in muffin trays.
6. Bake in oven for 20 to 23 minutes.
7. Place frittatas on cooling rack before serving.

## Baked Bean Quesadillas

Preparation Time: 35 minutes

Serves: 12

Ingredients:

- 1 tablespoon vegetable oil
- 1 onion, finely chopped
- 2 cloves garlic, minced
- 1 green pepper, chopped
- 2 tomatoes, chopped
- 140 grams frozen sweet corn
- 12 flour tortillas
- 415 grams Discovery Refried Beans
- 110 grams cheddar cheese, grated

Instructions:

1. Preheat oven to 190C.
2. In a frying pan, heat 1 tablespoon oil over medium fire. Stir in onion and garlic and sauté until onion is tender.
3. Add pepper, tomatoes and sweet corn. Stir until cooked.
4. Spread vegetable mixture over a tortilla. Add refried beans. Top with grated cheese. Cover with another tortilla to make a sandwich.
5. Bake for 10 to 15 minutes or until cheese has melted and tortillas are light brown.

## Grilled Aubergine and Stir-Fried Vegetables

Ready In: 30 minutes

Serves: 4

Ingredients:

- 1 aubergine
- 1 to 2 teaspoons vegetable oil
- 1 medium onion, chopped
- 2 plum tomatoes, chopped
- 1/4 teaspoon ground cayenne pepper
- Salt and black pepper
- 4 sprigs coriander, chopped

Instructions:

1. Preheat the oven grill. Place aubergine on a rack and grill for 5 minutes or until half the skin is burned.
2. Transfer aubergine to a microwave-safe dish. Set the microwave to a setting of high and let the aubergine cook for 5 minutes.
3. Take out aubergine and set aside to cool.
4. Peel off the skin, leaving on a few bits of burnt skin. Slice the aubergine into thick lengthwise pieces.
5. In a frying pan, heat vegetable oil over medium heat. Cook onion in oil until tender. Stir in tomatoes and aubergine. Flavor with cayenne pepper, salt and black pepper. Continue cooking until aubergine is soft and tender.

6. Take out from heat. Garnish with coriander.

## Beetroot, Orange and Apple Salad

Preparation Time: 40 minutes

Serves: 4

Ingredients:

- 675 grams beetroots, greens set aside
- 1 large orange
- 2 Granny Smith apples, peeled, cored and sliced
- 1 tablespoon olive oil
- 1 tablespoon raspberry vinegar
- 1/2 teaspoon caster sugar
- 1/4 teaspoon salt
- 1 clove garlic, minced
- 2 tablespoons toasted sunflower seeds, unsalted

Instructions:

1. Wash beetroots and dry.
2. Cut beetroot greens and set aside.
3. Cover beetroots in a saucepan with water and boil. Place the lid on and reduce heat. Let beetroots simmer for 20 minutes or until they're tender.
4. Drain and cool. Peel beetroots and cut into long slices.
5. Peel orange and section.
6. In a large mixing bowl, combine beetroots, oranges and apples.
7. Combine olive oil, raspberry vinegar, sugar and salt and pepper in a separate bowl.

8. Pour dressing over beetroot mixture and toss.
9. Arrange beetroot greens on a salad plate. Place beetroot salad over greens. Sprinkled with toasted sunflower seeds and serve.

## Black Bean Cakes

Preparation Time: 1 hour, 25 minutes

Serves: 12

Ingredients:

- 500 grams dried black turtle beans
- 1 tablespoon ground cumin
- 1/2 teaspoon chili powder
- 1 teaspoon cornmeal
- 1 egg
- 1/2 teaspoon salt
- Fresh coriander, chopped

For Cake Sauce:

- 8 tablespoons low-fat plain yoghurt
- 1 tablespoon semi-skimmed milk
- 1 pinch cayenne pepper

Instructions:

1. In a large pot, cover black beans with water and boil. Reduce heat and let simmer for one hour or until beans are tender.
2. Place cooked beans in a food processor and blend until smooth. Add cumin, chili powder, cornmeal, egg, salt and coriander and blend.
3. Take 3 tablespoons of black beans mixture and roll into a ball. Place baked bean ball between two

sheets of grease-free baking paper and press until flattened to discs as thick as your finger.

4. Repeat until all the mixture has been flattened.
5. In a large frying pan, heat oil over medium fire.
6. Cook black bean cakes, allowing 2 to 3 minutes for each side.
7. Sauce Recipe:
8. Mix yoghurt, semi-skimmed milk and cayenne pepper and stir.
9. Drizzle over black bean cakes while still hot.

# Dinner Recipes

## Braised Lamb, Green Beans and Tomatoes

Preparation Time: 1 hour, 20 minutes

Serves: 6

Ingredients:

- 600 grams lamb stewing meat
- 1 kilogram fresh green beans, washed and trimmed
- 600 grams passata
- 1 tablespoon olive oil
- 1 large red onion, chopped
- 225 ml water
- Salt and black pepper
- 1 dessertspoon fresh mint leaves, chopped

Instructions:

1. In a large frying pan, heat oil over medium to high heat.
2. Stir in onions and lamb meat. Cook until meat is brown.
3. Add green beans and cook for 10 minutes. Stir occasionally.
4. Add passata, water, salt, pepper and mint.
5. Reduce to low fire and place the lid.
6. Let the mixture simmer for one hour or until beans are tender.

7. Serve over long grain rice or pasta cooked al dente.

Tips:

If the mixture is watery, remove the lid and simmer for the remaining 30 minutes.

## American-Style Baked Beans

Preparation Time: 1 hour, 25 minutes

Serves: 8

Ingredients:

- 6 pieces bacon
- 1 medium onion, chopped
- 1 clove garlic, crushed
- 400 grams canned baked beans
- 400 grams canned borlotti beans
- 400 grams canned cannellini beans, drained
- 400 grams canned red kidney beans, drained
- 400 grams canned chickpeas, drained
- 3/4 cup tomato sauce
- 1/2 cup treacle
- 2 tablespoons Worcestershire sauce
- 4 tablespoons brown sugar
- 1 tablespoon French mustard
- 1/2 teaspoon black pepper

Instructions:

1. Preheat oven to 190C.
2. Cook bacon in a large frying pan. Drain, leaving 2 tablespoons of bacon drippings untouched.
3. Crush bacon into small pieces and place in a large bowl.
4. Place onion and garlic in the frying pan and cook in leftover bacon drippings until onion is tender.

Drain and add onion and garlic to the crushed bacon.

5. Add baked beans, borlotti beans, cannellini beans, red kidney beans and chickpeas.
6. Mix in tomato sauce, treacle, Worcestershire sauce, French mustard, brown sugar and black pepper. Fold mixture until well-blended.
7. Transfer the mixture into an oven-proof dish and cover.
8. Bake for 1 hour. Best served warm.

## Barley and Mushrooms with Cannellini Beans

Ready In: 1 hour, 15 minutes

Serves: 6

Ingredients:

- 1 teaspoon olive oil
- 225 grams sliced fresh mushrooms
- 2 medium onions, chopped
- 1 stalk celery, chopped
- 2 cloves garlic, minced
- 90 grams uncooked pearl barley
- 750 ml, vegetable stock
- 400 grams cannellini beans, drained

Instructions:

1. In a saucepan, heat olive oil over medium heat. Add mushrooms, onion, celery and garlic. Stir-fry until soft.
2. Add vegetable stock and barley into the mixture. Boil, cover and reduce heat.
3. Let the mixture simmer for 45 to 50 minutes to allow barley to become tender.
4. Add beans and let the mixture simmer for another 5 minutes or until the beans are cooked.

## Beef and Barley Soup

Preparation Time: 1 hour, 35 minutes

Serves: 6

Ingredients:

- 2 liters beef stock
- 200 grams cooked beef, sliced
- 340 grams pearl barley
- Black pepper

Instructions:

1. Pour beef stock into a large pot and boil.
2. Add beef and barley. Cover pot and let the mixture simmer for one hour.
3. Add freshly ground black pepper to taste.
4. Let the soup sit until it thickens to desired consistency.

Tips:

If too much water evaporates, add a few more cups.

## Fig and Lemon Chicken

Preparation Time: 55 minutes

Serves: 12

Ingredients:

- 12 chicken thighs
- 675 grams dried figs
- 1 lemon, juiced
- 1 lemon, peeled and sliced
- 3 tablespoons dark brown soft sugar
- 4 tablespoons white wine vinegar
- 4 tablespoons water
- Salt and pepper
- 1 handful fresh parsley, chopped

Instructions:

1. Preheat oven to 200C.
2. Combine lemon juice, vinegar, water and brown sugar in a small bowl. Stir until sugar is moist. Set aside.
3. Line the bottom of a large baking dish with figs and lemon slices. Put chicken thighs on top. Drizzle lemon juice mixture over the chicken and add salt and pepper to taste.
4. Bake in oven for 40 to 50 minutes or until juices run clear. Turn figs if they become brown. Baste chicken frequently.
5. Remove chicken, figs and lemon from baking pan and arrange on a platter.

6. Remove fat from cooking juices and drizzle over chicken.
7. Garnish with fresh parsley before serving.

# Penne with Tomatoes, Cannellini Beans and Feta Cheese

Preparation Time: 25 minutes

Serves: 4

Ingredients:

- 500 grams penne pasta
- 400 grams chopped tomatoes
- 400 grams cannellini beans
- 200 grams feta cheese, crumbled
- 300 grams fresh spinach, chopped

Instructions:

1. Cook pasta in a saucepan of boiling water until al dente. Drain and set aside.
2. In a large frying pan, heat tomatoes and cannellini beans and bring to a boil. Let mixture simmer for 10 minutes.
3. Add spinach to the sauce and cook until spinach is wilted. Stir constantly.
4. Pour the sauce over pasta and scatter feta over sauce generously.

## Quinoa Pilaf

Preparation Time: 35 minutes

Serves: 4

Ingredients:

- 175 grams uncooked quinoa
- 450 ml vegetable stock
- 1 tablespoon butter, unsalted
- 4 cloves garlic, chopped
- 2 sprigs thyme, stems removed
- 1 small onion, chopped,
- 1/4 teaspoon salt
- 1 handful fresh parsley, chopped
- 1 tablespoon lemon juice (optional)

Instructions:

1. In a saucepan, heat butter until melted over medium fire. Stir in quinoa and toast for 5 minutes or until quinoa turns a light brown color. Stir occasionally.
2. Add vegetable stock and bring to a boil. Cover saucepan and reduce heat to a simmer. Cook for 15 minutes or until quinoa is soft.
3. Mix garlic, thyme, onion, parsley and salt in a large mixing bowl.
4. Add the quinoa and mix.
5. Drizzle a bit of lemon juice if desired and serve.

## Balsamic Steak with Tomato Pasta Salad

Preparation Time: 1 hour, 15 minutes

Serves: 4

Ingredients:

- 200 grams penne pasta, dried
- 4 150-gram beef sirloin steaks
- 250 grams cherry truss tomatoes
- 2 tablespoons olive oil
- 1/4 cup balsamic vinegar
- 2 cloves garlic, crushed
- 1/4 cup fresh basil leaves
- 50 grams baby rocket
- Olive oil cooking spray

Instructions:

1. Cook pasta in a saucepan of boiling water until al dente. Drain and add 1 tablespoon olive oil, then toss.
2. In a large glass bowl, mix vinegar, olive oil and 1/2 clove garlic. Place steak pieces and let sit in marinade for several minutes.
3. Spray cooking oil on a char-grill and heat over medium to high heat.
4. Grill steaks for 3 to 4 minutes on each side for medium, less for rare and more for well-done.
5. Place steaks on a plate and cover with foil.
6. Grill tomatoes for 2 to 3 minutes or until cooked to your liking.

7. Mix tomatoes, basil and baby rocket to pasta. Toss to combine.
8. Serve steaks over pasta salad.

# Dessert Recipes

## No-Bake Pineapple and Berry Cheesecake

Preparation Time: 4 hours, 30 minutes

Serves: 10

Ingredients:

- 3 cups light cream cheese
- 2 cups non-fat cream cheese
- 4 cups vanilla ice cream cones, crushed
- 5 sheets leaf gelatin
- 2 tablespoons powdered milk
- 2 teaspoons vanilla essence
- 1 1/2 cups canned pineapple
- 1 1/2 cups strawberries, halved
- 1/2 cup fresh blueberries

Instructions:

1. Soften gelatin by soaking in cold water for five minutes.
2. Combine 1/2 cup non-fat cream cheese and crushed ice cream cones and mix with your fingers. Layer the mixture at the bottom of a spring form pan. Pack the crust tightly and place in refrigerator.
3. Drain pineapple, reserving the juice for later use. Cut into small chunks and set aside.

4. Place remaining non-fat cream cheese, light cream cheese, vanilla essence and powdered milk in a large mixing bowl. Stir and mix.
5. Drain the gelatin and place in a saucepan over low fire. Pour in the juice from the canned pineapple and stir.
6. Pour the gelatin mixture into the cream cheese mixture slowly. Stir frequently.
7. Add the pineapple chunks to the cream cheese.
8. Take out the crust from the refrigerator and cover with cream cheese. Arrange strawberries and blueberries on top and place in refrigerator again. Let cool for four hours before serving.

## Orange Passion Fruit Custards

Preparation Time: 35 minutes

Serves: 4

Ingredients:

- 2 passion fruits, halved
- 2 teaspoons orange rind, finely grated
- 1 tablespoon custard powder
- 1 cup low-fat milk
- 3 eggs, lightly beaten
- 1/4 cup caster sugar

Instructions:

1. Preheat oven to 180C.
2. Blend custard powder and milk until smooth. Mix in eggs, sugar, passion fruit and orange rind and mix well.
3. Pour mixture into oven-proof ramekins.
4. Place ramekins in a deep baking pan. Pour water into pan until half of the ramekins are submerged.
5. Baked for 20 to 25 minutes or until custards are set.

## Pear Chocolate Fudge Cake

Preparation Time: 1 hour

Serves: 12

Ingredients:

- 1 cup plain wholegrain flour
- 1/2 cup raw almonds, ground
- 1/4 cup semolina
- 1/4 cup rye flour
- 2 pears, unskinned and grated
- 1 pear, sliced thinly
- 3/4 cup skim milk
- 1/2 cup olive oil
- 2 eggs
- 200 grams dark chocolate
- 1 teaspoon vanilla essence
- 1 tablespoon liqueur
- 1 teaspoon bicarbonate soda

For topping:

- 50 grams dark chocolate
- 1/2 cup coconut, shredded

Instructions:

1. Preheat oven to 180C.
2. Lightly grease a spring form cake pan or lamington tin.

3. Break 200 grams chocolate and place in a heat-proof bowl. Place bowl in a saucepan filled with water up to the lower half of the bowl. Bring water to a boil to melt the chocolate.
4. Sift flours into a mixing bowl and add almonds and semolina.
5. In another bowl, whisk eggs and milk until smooth. Stir in vanilla essence, oil and liqueur. Add bicarbonate soda and baking powder and mix gently.
6. Pour liquid mixture into dry ingredients. Add grated pears and mix. Pour 3/4 of melted chocolate and mix.
7. Place batter into spring form cake pan and spread evenly. Insert a toothpick in the center and bake for 30 to 45 minutes or until toothpick comes out clean.
8. Let the cake cool for 10 minutes.
9. Apply the remaining melted chocolate on the surface and sides of the cake. Arrange sliced pears on top for decorate and sprinkle grated coconut over the pears.

# Like this book?

Thanks for purchasing and reading this book. I'm positive that if you just follow the GI diet, you will reach your weight loss goals a lot easier and quicker than you realize.

However, could you spare one minute and do me a quick favour though?

Could you write a little review on Amazon about this book?

I love getting feedback and knowing I'm helping people makes a real difference to me. I read all my reviews and would really appreciate your thoughts.

Just visit the website address below to leave your comments:

http://bit.ly/gibelly

Thanks again and I wish you the best of luck.

Wesley Atkins

**DISCLAIMER AND/OR LEGAL NOTICES:** Every effort has been made to accurately represent this book and it's potential. Results vary with every individual, and your results may or may not be different from those depicted. No promises, guarantees or warranties, whether stated or implied, have been made that you will produce any specific result from the "Low GI Belly Fat Diet". Your efforts are individual and unique, and may vary from those shown. Your success depends on your efforts, background and motivation.

The material in this publication is provided for educational and informational purposes only and is not intended as medical advice. The information contained in this book should not be used to diagnose or treat any illness, metabolic disorder, disease or health problem. Always consult your physician or health care provider before beginning any nutrition or exercise program. Use of the programs, advice, and information contained in this book is at the sole choice and risk of the reader.

Printed in Great Britain
by Amazon